NNG's Formula to Kick Cramp's Ass!

A blueprint to naturally get rid of menstrual cramps

Brittany Walker

ISBN:

      Paperback: 979-8-9862279-0-0
      E-Book: 979-8-9862279-1-7
      Audiobook: 979-8-9862279-2-4

Edited by: Abigail McIntosh
Formatted by: Accuracy 4 Sure
Designed by: NNG Publishing
Photography Credit: NNG Publishing, Vagesty, LLC & Canva, Inc.

This is a publication based on real case studies, statistics and years of research by the author - a Plant-Based Nutritionist, former Biology Professor and retired Chef.

Disclaimer. All of the recommendations are solely based on the author's personal and client's case studies, research, and proven testimonies. The author is not a licensed medical physician however is a proficient nutritionist who has and continues to experience no cramps each menstrual cycle by following these suggestions. This methodology may not work for you however it has been a successful resource for the author, and she shares it with you in the hopes to help you as well.

Dedication

To all the women tired of the shit that menstruation puts us through! This one is for you, Goddess! Also, to the Gods supporting the women in their lives (lovers, mothers, sisters or daughters) - we appreciate you taking time to educate yourself to help heal us.

"What you put in and/or on your body determines the REAL path to *The Fountain of Youth!*"

— Brittany Walker

Foreword

Aunt Flow. End of a sentence. The Red Sea. Time of the month. Red-headed stepchild. Period. Menstrual cycle.

Ladies, no matter what you call it, we instinctively know what it means. For some, it's an easy, breezy kind of week. For the unfortunate ones, it's a time of excruciating pain, nausea, hot/cold flashes, days in bed, heavy and uncontrollable bleeding, plus so much more. When I first met Brittany (I call her "B"), she caught me at the end of a clinical study that I participated in 2013. The study was on the effects of a new medication that targeted extremely severe menstrual cramps; a portion of the individuals had placebos, whilst the other group had the real medicine. During the study, I KNEW I had gotten the "real deal"; my cramps lessened, and I was no longer nauseous.

About 4 months after the study, all conditions resurfaced in full force stating, "Hey! We missed you!" For years, I dealt with these crippling symptoms, and fast forward to 2015, I joined the Army; I took this opportunity to seek professional assistance and determine if there was anything the doctors could do to ease the enfeebling pains. Their only solution? *800mg ibuprofen*. That was the cure-all, know-all medicine of choice. It "cured" everything, or so they think.

Many moons later, I reached out to Brittany to see if she knew any natural or holistic methods that would help a sistah out! I was the first person to discover that B had Diabetes after she was diagnosed in 2014. Knowing her history with extensive negative medical outcomes, overcoming abuse, and transitioning to a plant-based lifestyle to save herself, and others; I put my faith in her. She always has had the passion to serve, heal, educate, and I knew she would work effortlessly to restore my body as she has done with so many individuals over the last decade.

That is when she hit me with the Holy Grail! Turmeric, ginger, cinnamon, high-quality h2o, herbal teas, controlling my body temperature, soaking in the tub, monitoring my food intake, and yoni steams. All of these factors collectively contribute to the formula she created to *kick my cramp's ass*! Being hard-headed and stationed across the world in South Korea, I pushed this legitimate and proven formula to the back of my mind. I returned to the United States still doing the tango with menstrual cramps.

It was not until March 2021 that I decided I needed to change something, and with B's help, I succeeded! I finally heeded her advice. There was a point where I was severely nauseous and constantly vomiting for three days; I could not eat or drink anything! B took it upon herself to send me what I call "The Green Juice." Although it was not my cup of tea, I drank it. From that day forward, I followed everything she told me to do. I began to add ginger, turmeric and cinnamon to my hot tea, and food.

In April 2021, I stopped eating meat and went vegan cold turkey! With B being a retired chef and restaurateur, and having an extreme love for southern, soul and Cajun food, then I could give up what I had been conditioned to eat my entire life. When we know better, we do better... right?! Not even three weeks in, my body was positively changing; three days of pain went down to two!

By June 2021, I went from being in severe pain with PMS symptoms for multiple days to only one day! Cutting out unhealthy foods like soda, sweets and meat made a drastic difference to my overall health. Alcohol was never something I drank regularly, so giving that the boot was uncomplicated. I know many people struggle to give up alcohol, and it's understandable with how it's projected in society. I used to enjoy a Whiskey Sour and when B told me she cut alcohol out altogether, (and boy did she love her *Maker's Mark* Manhattans, Whiskey Sours or a Pinor Noir), I knew it was the right move for me.

At last, I was starting to see light at the end of the tunnel, and like a thief in the night, I got sick. The nausea during my cycle would induce vomiting, and I could not seem to shake it. Instructed by my superiors, I had to go back to the doctor for an examination. Upon testing, and receiving a pelvic ultrasound, they discovered a tumor in my cervix. My entire world came to a halt; the tumor would enlarge during my cycle causing intense cramps, heavy bleeding, nausea, and vomiting. Their solution? Birth control. Again, the only recommended resolution for my uterine health issues was medication. Becoming vegan meant I no longer wanted to consume chemicals. Since age 19, I have been tossing back 800mg ibuprofen once a month to find relief, and after 16 years I have had enough! I went back to the drawing board with B and enhanced my regimen. We were determined to *kick cramp's ass*!

Being stricter with my diet, cutting out processed foods, drinking plenty of water, receiving ample amounts of rest, paying close attention to my body, switching from tampons to the *Flex* menstrual disc, incorporating yoni steams into my routine, using *The HoneyPot Co* feminine wash, not drinking alcohol, and ensuring I was adding greens, turmeric, and ginger to my daily intake made a world of a difference in my life. Brittany made a difference in my life!

By simply following her formula, I began to find the relief I heard her describe. When she told me she was going to share this awareness in a book; I knew immediately that the world needed this information. Knowing she has always had my best interest at heart, I trusted her, and like a star in the fourth quarter, she rose to the challenge, and hit the game-winning shot! B is an example of someone who overcame addiction, substance abuse, chronic illnesses, and mental disease. Sharing her methods, and knowledge has always been a part of who she is as she is keen to galvanize. She is a true alchemist, healer, and educator! I am very proud of her, and this book! In reading this, I hope that you find the strength to make the applicable changes to conquer your wellness, and understand the journey may be hard, but the final, lifelong results are well worth it!

—SGT J. Williams, *CBRN Specialist* - **United States Army**

x

Table of Contents

Introduction

"Menstrual pain was reported by 84.1% of women, with 43.1% reporting that pain occurred during every period, and 41% reporting that pain occurred during some periods." Grandi, G., Ferrari, S., Xholli, A., Cannoletta, M., Palma, F., Romani, C., Volpe, A., & Cagnacci, A. (2012)[1]

If you have not heard it yet, your womb is DIVINE! You MUST treat it with an abundance of care - that's what makes you POWERFUL! It is the most sacred space you possess; it is up to you, Goddess to nurture your womb and protect it from factors that will slowly destroy the essential part of a women's health. Once you can grasp this concept then you are on the golden route to achieving optimal health.

I could hear the harps playing and the angels singing, because at that very moment, I discovered what causes a cramp-free body! After suffering from a strenuous history of menstrual cycles, this has been one of my greatest accomplishments thus far. Years of detailed case studies, research, and analytics has led to the formula that relieves pain and inflammation from what some call *Code Red*. **DEATH TO DYSMENORRHEA!** It is considered taboo to discuss our menstrual cycles at any age as a woman in our culture, but we are here

---

[1] Grandi, G., Ferrari, S., Xholli, A., Cannoletta, M., Palma, F., Romani, C., Volpe, A., & Cagnacci, A. (2012). Prevalence of menstrual pain in young women: what is dysmenorrhea?. *Journal of pain research*, 5, 169–174. https://doi.org/10.2147/JPR.S30602

to bust the gates wide open with normalizing the necessary discussions. Just to think where we all would be if we had a blueprint on how to conquer dealing with this monthly madness labeled as menstruation.

Not like the current average age of starting a menstrual cycle at 12 years-old (in the 90's), I was one month away from turning 15 years-old when my cycle started during my 5th period class of my freshman year of high school. After a traumatic sexual encounter, I started my first period within 24 hours and assumed the pain was from the incident. As the women in my family called it, I had encountered "the hereditary curse" of the menstrual cycle. I distinctly remember my T-Lady (Top Lady, aka your mother in Texas) being out of town, and my brother, who was a freshman in college, walked to my best friend's house to get me some pads because he did not want to walk around the store with feminine hygiene products. I never understood that about young men because you cannot use any of the products! That helped for a bit but being the Daddy's Girl that I am, I called Papa Bear before he was heading home from work. He literally walked in the house with several Wal-Mart bags full of pads, tampons, panty liners, and cramp medication with ibuprofen only. I am allergic to acetaminophen and the stronger pain relievers are acetaminophen based. Pain medications and heating pads were the answer for the next few years. At 21, my OB/GYN introduced the idea of birth control in order to "regulate" my cycle. I tried a few different forms of birth control and various doses because I kept experiencing adverse reactions, which added to the already heavy PMS symptoms.

Throughout my 20's, I was diagnosed with various illnesses associated with both my physical and mental health. This led to being prescribed with multiple medications all within a small time frame. In addition, I was in my young, rebellious stage so I was engaging in a lifestyle that was unhealthy and causing unbalanced chemical reactions.

At this point, I could not keep up with my cycle as some months it would be 1 week, and others it would be 14 days. While I may have cramped heavily for 5 days consecutively one month with a light flow, the following month, I would cramp heavily for 3 days with an extremely heavy flow. It was torture and I began to dread each month because I had absolutely no control over my menstruation. Without having a synchronized schedule, I was not provided a warning when my cycle was starting, which also became frustrating.

In 2011, I stopped taking birth control because I read an article about how there may have been an association with having trouble getting pregnant once you were ready to conceive with specific brands. Why is birth control, which has the potential to lead to infertility, be the only recommendation?! Researching this information in detail gave me vibes from when my ancestors were experimented on during slavery or the Tuskegee Study. Feels like population control but that is a different story. Eliminating birth control aided in easing some of my PMS symptoms, such as having a more consistent cycle of only 5-7 days each month, and only cramping during the first 3 days. However, the pain and the flow were still hindering my day-to-day activities. I would plan my PTO (Paid Time Off) around my cycle so that I could have the first 2 days to hibernate on the heating pad, take meds, and bundle up. Being allergic to acetaminophen did not leave many over-the-counter options that were strong enough to handle my tolerance. So, the prescribed medication 800-1000mg kept me lackadaisical; therefore, I preferred not to work during these times. This went on for 6 years.

A major life event was scheduled for the end of 2017, which led me to dropping some pounds. During the past few years, I gained an excessive amount of weight and was attempting different workout plans in order to meet my desired goal. I could not seem to gain any progress by losing 10 pounds here and there, then gaining it back instantly. 88 days before the event, "What the Health?" on Netflix was recommended to me to gain some additional knowledge on different lifestyles. After the credits came to an end, I was flabbergasted, mouth wide opened and completely baffled at what I realistically had been consuming my entire life. That was 8/13/2017 and my life changed forever as I transitioned to a Vegan lifestyle cold turkey. I immediately threw everything away in my refrigerator and pantry that was not made from plants. The scientist in me began to record the various changes that I was making. In September 2017, I stopped taking medication for cramps and inflammation.

Over the next year, I noticed drastic transformations with the lifestyle adjustments that had been made. I knew that I was onto something life changing; not only for myself, but other women who suffer from the same symptoms. I also returned to school and graduated with a Master of Science in Nutrition Education.

By July 2019, I had experimented with different techniques consistently notating and abiding by the factors that showcased significant improvements. Although I was 80% sure of how to eliminate menstrual cramps and decrease PMS symptoms. I would still fluctuate months where I would cramp for 1 or 2 days; or I could not control my temperature, which led to excruciating convulsions. I had come this far and refused to give up on what truly can cause the body to get rid of these tiresome pains.

Some of my favorite resources during this period were "African Holistic Health" by Llaila Afrika, and "Heal Thyself for Health and Longevity" and "Sacred Woman" by Queen Afua. The techniques presented in each literature further confirmed multiple hypotheses I had formulated. Many holistic methodologies led to not only reversing cramps but also preventing and eliminating other uterine health diagnoses, including

PMS symptoms, endometriosis, fibroids, Polycystic Ovary Syndrome (PCOS) and infertility.

I decided to go on an alcohol cleanse and engage in a fitness challenge for 30 days. Although I had worked out since transitioning my diet, it was never a consistent routine that lasted longer than a 2-week period. I extended the alcohol cleanse to 52 days, then after a 2-week period eliminated alcohol from my diet completely. As for physical activity, I worked my way up to exercising Monday-Friday at a minimum of 40 minutes per day. Then I incorporated additional changes to my nutrition such as sea moss and decreasing "junk" Vegan food with Plant-Based items as a replacement.

After a couple of months of the new changes, my cramps diminished; ecstatic was an understatement! Before I shared my remedies and tips, I wanted to ensure this was a solid algorithm. I evaluated a significant amount of data over the next 1.5-years throughout this 5-year experiment, and still produced the same results. At that point, I knew it was time to share how others could kick cramp's ass! So, let's get into this kick ass formula.

Chapter 1

Prologue (aka My Helpful Tips)

"Dysmenorrhea seems to be associated with late or early menarche, prolonged and heavier than normal menstrual flow, low body weight and body mass index, inadequate physical exercise, genetic predisposition, active and passive cigarette smoking, low socioeconomic status, diet, stress, and mental illness." Grandi, G., Ferrari, S., Xholli, A., Cannoletta, M., Palma, F., Romani, C., Volpe, A., & Cagnacci, A. (2012)[2]

Before outlining the exact steps I take to ensure a painless menstrual cycle, I would like to provide some helpful tips. Setting the expectations is key and will ultimately help you if you choose to go on this journey:

1. Be **PATIENT**! Hard work pays off and this is not a fast journey. Most individuals want instant gratification but when you transition to holistic practices, the natural route takes longer than expected. We must be realistic that it took years for these symptoms and diagnoses to develop; so, it will take time to reverse the damage. It

---

[2] Grandi, G., Ferrari, S., Xholli, A., Cannoletta, M., Palma, F., Romani, C., Volpe, A., & Cagnacci, A. (2012). Prevalence of menstrual pain in young women: what is dysmenorrhea?. *Journal of pain research*, *5*, 169–174. https://doi.org/10.2147/JPR.S30602

took me a year to reduce symptoms significantly so speaking of the #2 tip...

2. **TRUST** the process! When doubt or fear surfaces be sure to stay positive and remember there is a greater prize for following through with your plan of action. Every woman's body is different so the time it may take for the formula to start working will vary by case.

3. **SOAK** up some sun! The natural form of vitamin D will aid in not only, regulating your body temperature, but providing your body with nutrients that will improve your pain, mood and managing body weight.

4. Be Mindful of **MEDICATIONS**! I did not take any medication for over 2 years before my cramps completely went away. Be aware that if you are on prescribed medication, the ingredients may be contributing to cramps and inflammation.

5. Stay **HYDRATED**! The more water, tea and freshly squeezed juice you consume during your cycle, the better as it reduces discomfort and PMS symptoms by replenishing the fluids that the body is releasing.

6. I am **NOT** a doctor! However, I am a Plant-Based Nutritionist, former Biology Professor and retired Chef, who lives by this formula, and it works for me! If you have pre-existing

diagnoses, I can understand your concerns so practice what you feel most comfortable with.

7. **AVOID** foods that are processed, have added sugars and salt! These ingredients and methods aid in developing inflammation, and PMS symptoms in the body.

8. **DECREASE** your caffeine intake! Eliminate food, beverages, pain relievers or supplements that contain caffeine. Caffeine increases estrogen levels which activates PMS symptoms due to a hormone blockage narrowing the blood vessels, therefore, increases inflammation.

9. **FOCUS** on taking deep breaths when you feel the pain emerging! Breathing exercises are essential for cramps. Take a deep breath in, hold for 3 seconds, then take 3 seconds blowing it out. Repeat until the pain decreases to a manageable level.

10. Be **MINDFUL** of how frequently you are changing your underwear! The sweat and bodily fluids retained in the material aids in your overall vaginal health. I recommend eliminating underwear when you feel comfortable, and you will notice that when you allow *Her* to breathe, you will experience less negative menstrual symptoms each month.

11. Do not forget to **STRETCH**! Partaking in yoga moves for a minimum of 15 minutes every other day can help decrease cramp pain and other PMS symptoms. Fluid movement like dancing or serenading your divinity in the mirror and showing absolute love for yourself is essential!

12. **ELIMINATE** all forms of chemicals and toxins from entering your body! This includes the food, beverages, toiletries and household items that you are currently utilizing. Even if the ingredients show a small amount of chemicals, a small amount overtime will lead to a larger problem such as a diagnosis or chronic illness.

13. Do **NOT** **QUIT**! This is not an easy walk in the park, but it is definitely worth it. There will be times when you want to give up but overcoming the obstacles will supersede the desire to quit. Stay disciplined; this is not an easy journey, and it takes focus and consistency to achieve it. The time to become the best YOU is now! Take full accountability of the information that you acquire and use this to your advantage! Once you overcome the obstacles of transitions, everything will be a smooth evolution.

Chapter 2

NNG's Kick Ass Formula

- ☀ **Iron Levels: 7 Days Prior to Starting**

- ☀ **Ginger: Daily**

- ☀ **Turmeric: Daily**

- ☀ **Herbs: Daily**

- ☀ **Spices: Daily**

- ☀ **Yoni Steams: Annually**

- ☀ **Period Tracking: Monthly**

- ☀ **Temperature Control: 2 Days Prior and During**

- ☀ **Hot Bath Soak: Twice Weekly**

- ☀ **Organic Feminine Hygiene Products: Daily and As Needed**

- ☀ **Plant-Based Diet: Daily**

- ☀ **Physical Activity: Minimum 5x Weekly at Minimum of 40 Minutes Daily**

- ☀ **No Alcohol**

Chapter 3

The World's Leading Deficiency

"Among women of reproductive age, menstrual blood loss is the most common cause of ID and IDA." (Fernandez-Jimenez, Moreno, Wright, Shih, Vaquero & Remacha, 2020)[3]

Iron happens to be the most prominent nutrient deficiency across the globe. Although red meat and eggs are recommended as sources of iron, one may potentially think the deficit would not be at an all-time high. Iron is an essential micronutrient needed for developmental growth; primarily to aid in transporting oxygen throughout the body. This mineral makes hemoglobin, a protein in the red blood cells, and is also used to produce hormones in the body. Your iron levels decrease as you lose blood each month. If you are not adequately replacing the lost iron, this can lead to iron anemia. Low levels of this nutrient may lead to being extremely fatigued, inflammation, weakness, or feeling cold. Some of these symptoms are identical to PMS so

[3] Fernandez-Jimenez MC, Moreno G, Wright I, Shih PC, Vaquero MP, Remacha AF. Iron Deficiency in Menstruating Adult Women: Much More than Anemia. Women's Health Rep (New Rochelle). 2020;1(1):26-35. Published 2020 Jan 29. doi:10.1089/whr.2019.0011

it is imperative that we acquire a legitimate amount as frequently as possible.

Why not get ahead of the game by maintaining a positive level of iron, versus suffering after the damage is already done?

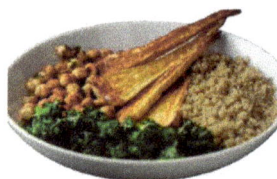

☀ **NNG recommends increasing your iron intake 7 days leading up to your cycle.**

This is providing the body with enough iron to replace what will be lost. Plant forms of iron tend to provide an adequate source that is organic and free of genetically modified objects (GMOs), toxins or chemicals. The foods packed with iron that have been frequent in my diet are:

- ⊙ Quinoa (throw some herbs and spices to give it some flavor!)
- ⊙ Chickpeas (Garbanzo beans)
- ⊙ Teff (Injera bread from an authentic Ethiopian restaurant is our favorite!)
- ⊙ Seeds (hemp, pumpkin and chia)
- ⊙ Leafy Greens (Collard, Kale, Spinach)
- ⊙ Legumes (lentils, whole grains, beans, peas)
- ⊙ Nuts (walnuts, cashews, pecans)
- ⊙ Mushrooms (preferably chopped or minced so it can fold easily into a recipe)

- Berries (elderberries, raspberries, blackberries, blueberries and strawberries)

"Education is the passport to the future, for tomorrow belongs to those who prepare for it today." — Malcolm X

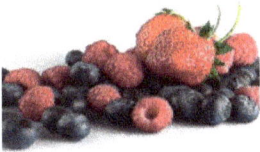

To take it a step further, incorporate iron into your daily meals! This will aid in decreasing your cramps and assist with your overall health. It is vital to digest iron daily and this will be described in more detail in the section labeled *"Plant-Based Diet"*. The chlorophyll in leafy greens will not only boost your iron levels but also reduce inflammation, heavy bleeding and regulate moods. When your body has an adequate amount of iron once menstruation begins, the loss of blood will not tamper with your body temperature nor increase inflammation. If you notice that your inflammation is starting to kick in, then I recommend using a heating pad. I have been rocking the same heating pad ever since I started my cycle in 2000! It was originally my T-Lady's and she had it before I was born. Let's just say this vintage heating pad is still serving its purpose whenever I use it throughout the year. Now the hottest selection does not work anymore, however it still does the trick and has HERSTORY!

Chapter 4

My Detoxing Bestie

"Menstrual pain is a very common problem, but the need for medication and the inability to function normally occurs less frequently. Nevertheless, at least one in four women experiences distressing menstrual pain characterized by a need for medication and absenteeism from study or social activities." Grandi, G., Ferrari, S., Xholli, A., Cannoletta, M., Palma, F., Romani, C., Volpe, A., & Cagnacci, A. (2012)[4]

Ginger is a hidden gem that is vital for the human body! It has natural healing agents by reducing pain, bacteria, and inflammation within the body. The main bioactive compound is gingerol, which includes anti-inflammatory and antioxidant healing instruments; for your period, this means ginger can regulate the pain levels associated with Dysmenorrhea and help decrease heavy flows each month (Menorrhagia).

☀ **NNG recommends taking ginger on a daily basis.**

If you are unable to incorporate ginger into your daily routine, be sure to digest 3 days prior to your

[4] Grandi, G., Ferrari, S., Xholli, A., Cannoletta, M., Palma, F., Romani, C., Volpe, A., & Cagnacci, A. (2012). Prevalence of menstrual pain in young women: what is dysmenorrhea?. *Journal of pain research*, *5*, 169–174. https://doi.org/10.2147/JPR.S30602

period starting and during your period. This still gives the body enough time to activate and begin the regulating process. Below are the following ways that ginger is consumed in my diet:

- ⊙ In Food (I cook with it for every single meal)

- ⊙ Tea

- ⊙ Fresh Juices

- ⊙ Smoothies

- ⊙ Skin Products (cleanser, moisturizer, toner, etc.)

- ⊙ Other Beverages (Infused Water, Lemonades, Hot Cacao, etc.)

- ⊙ Wellness Shots

You will notice a significant difference once consuming ginger consistently. It assists with nausea, fighting infections, and lowers both blood sugar and cholesterol levels. With women, it is a staple for eliminating visceral fat (that stubborn belly skin) that we care for. During your period, while you may feel bloated, ginger can help reduce the unwanted weight gain for the short timeframe.

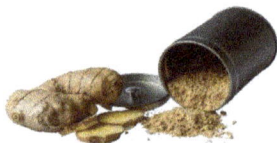

**"Healing has to be consistent with itself.
If it isn't then it is not healing. The
components have to be from life."
— Dr. Sebi**

It is imperative to detox the body frequently, freeing yourself of any built-up toxins or chemicals that may lead to developing issues. Ginger is *My Detoxing Bestie* because the cleansing results are worthwhile! Before I began these case studies, I would only consume ginger in Asian dishes, digesting the bestie at least once a week. The daily absorption has drastically enhanced my overall health and I encourage you to try it out!

Chapter 5

Living My Life Like It's GOLDEN

"Besides for relieving menstrual pain, curcumin [an active ingredient in turmeric) has many benefits. Research shows that curcumin helps in the oxidative and inflammatory conditions, metabolic syndrome, arthritis, anxiety, hyperlipidemia, improves recovery due to inflammation and muscle pain caused by exercise, and can provide other health benefits." (Rahman, Hardi, Maras & Riva, 2020).[5]

Turmeric possesses a bioactive compound named curcumin that aids in reducing inflammation in the body. It also aids in regulating hormones, controlling PMS symptoms, and stabilizing moods. Due to curcumin not being easily absorbed in the bloodstream, it is important to accompany it with other items such as black pepper that will assist during the absorption process. Now although this spice can stain everything in sight, it is a life saver and has done wonders for my overall optimal health.

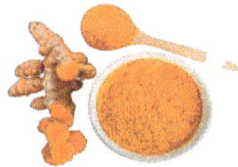

---

[5] Rahman, S. F., Hardi, G. W., Maras, M. A. J., and Riva, Y. R. (2020). Influence of Curcumin, and Ginger in Primary Dysmenorrhea: A Review. International Journal of Applied Engineering Research, 15(7), 634–638. Retrieved from www.ripublication.com.

☀ **NNG recommends consuming turmeric daily to activate its healing agents.**

A recognized anti-inflammatory promoter, it has more benefits and works more effectively than over-the-counter medication. Staying on top of your turmeric consumption will be a relief during your period, and if the body's immune system is weak. Below are the following ways that turmeric is consumed in my diet (similar to NNG's ginger regimen):

- ⊙ In Food (I cook with it for every single meal)
- ⊙ Tea
- ⊙ Fresh Juices
- ⊙ Smoothies
- ⊙ Skin Products (cleanser, moisturizer, toner, etc.)
- ⊙ Other Beverages (Infused Water, Lemonades, Hot Cacao, etc.)
- ⊙ Wellness Shots

"Sickness is the body's way of rebelling against disrespect and pollution."
— Queen Afua

Tip: Use a turmeric-based facial or skin product then sit in the sun! You divine supreme being... talk about radiate Goddess! That *Goddess Glow* is important for the neuromelanin we possess. Strutting down the beach, water hitting my feet, and *Naturaleza's Apothecary*'s *Show Your Glow* (contains turmeric) serum beaming off my face ignites a power within as I faintly hear Jill Scott singing, "Living my life like it's golden."

Chapter 6

Alchemy at Its Finest

"According to the World Health Organization, 75% of the world's populations are using herbs for basic healthcare needs." Pan, Litscher, Gao, Zhou, Yu, Chen, Zhang, Tang, Sun, & Ko. (2014)[6]

Herbal teas are natural antioxidants. The herbs aid in maintaining a healthy uterus; along with physical and mental health. Also, herbs decrease heavy bleeding (Menorrhagia), and inflammation. Most individuals might assume that you can only reap the benefits of herbs through tea, but you can also cook with them, use them for your yoni steams (detailed more in the section labeled *Womb Revitalization*), smoke them, or burn them in candles or incense. Acting as an anti-inflammatory, herbs also detoxifies the body, regulates hormones, and reduces stress.

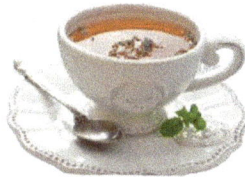

[6] Pan, S. Y., Litscher, G., Gao, S. H., Zhou, S. F., Yu, Z. L., Chen, H. Q., Zhang, S. F., Tang, M. K., Sun, J. N., & Ko, K. M. (2014). Historical perspective of traditional indigenous medical practices: the current renaissance and conservation of herbal resources. Evidence-based complementary and alternative medicine: eCAM, 2014, 525340. https://doi.org/10.1155/2014/525340

> ☀ **NNG recommends consuming herbs daily to rejuvenate the body as it aids in releasing toxins.**

Some of the herbs that NNG incorporates into the daily diet along with their benefits are:

- Burdock - reduces inflammation, frees toxins from the blood, antioxidants

- Calendula - eliminates bacterial vaginosis, decreases yeast infections, antioxidant, reduces discharge and bloating

- Chamomile - controls muscle spasms, antioxidant, decreases inflammation, regulates PMS symptoms, relieves anxiety, soothes nerves

- Chaste Tree - also known as Vitex boosts progesterone which regulates the estrogen

- Elderberry - anti-inflammatory, reduces pain, rich in antioxidants, disease fighting and prevention

- Green tea (decaffeinated) - reduces inflammation, improves blood flow, decreases bloating, increases water lost from the body

- Hibiscus - regulates menstruation, improves blood circulation, anti-inflammatory, regulates mood and other PMS symptoms

- ⊙ Motherwort - strengthens uterine muscles, decreases cramps, hormone regulator, encourages suppressed blood flow

- ⊙ Nettles - improves estrogen, regulates blood flow, mood regulator, packed with iron

- ⊙ Red Raspberry Leaf - tightens pelvic muscles, reduces muscles spasms, regulates PMS symptoms

- ⊙ Bay Leaves - reduces menstrual cramps, eliminates vaginal discharge, regulates blood flow and cycle duration

I am an avid tea lover! Try throwing all the above herbs into a loose-leaf diffuser combined with turmeric, ginger, cinnamon and black pepper. This is one of the best herbal infusions that manages your inflammation. If the mixture is too bitter for you, add dates, a healthy form of sweetener.

An alchemist is an individual who transforms situations for the better. With having the love for serving others, and healing people with holistic techniques, we strive to deliver alchemy at its finest! Funneled by Aja, (African Orisha of the woodland, its creatures, homegrown healers, and the first known woman alchemist), I am a firm believer in; 'the Earth has everything that we need to heal and cure ourselves naturally without the need of any chemical-based, toxic or man-made products'. Back in the 80's and 90's, if I cut myself then my Daddy would cut off a piece of aloe vera from his plant versus going to the drug store for ointment or over-the-counter medicine. If you feel a cough emerging, eat or drink fruits high in calcium and vitamin c with a mix of ginger and lemon. The stronger your immune system, the easier it will be to fight unwanted viruses, and illnesses. This is not stating that you will not feel any symptoms, however your body will naturally protect itself, and grow stronger as you increase adequate amounts and forms of macro and micro nutrients.

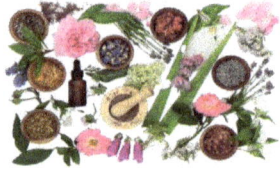

"Bringing the gifts that my ancestors gave, I am the dream and the hope of the slave." — Maya Angelou

When herbal techniques are mentioned, I am asked if cannabis/marijuana can be considered for alternative medicine. If it has natural (not man-made) seeds, can be grown, and have any added chemicals that are harmful to the body then yes, I consider this a substitute to over-the-counter or prescribed medicine constructed from harmful ingredients that strengthens unwanted diagnoses. Purchasing from a plant connoisseur who knows their strains is highly recommended to ensure tackling pain, inflammation or even mood swings versus being a humdrum couch potato. Indica will aid in supervising your pain levels, however sativa (my favorite!) will leave you focused and creative allowing you to still seize your day. Speaking to a budtender/budologist at your local dispensary can educate you on which flower they may have that is curated specifically for menstruation. If you reside in a state where cannabis is illegal, you should verify if the state is medicinal so you can satiate in Cannabidiol (CBD) options. CBD can be used in beverages, foods, salves, lotions, oils or even smoked. Back home in Texas, there is a melanin, women and veteran owned business called *Lazy Daze Tea* that has multiple options for hot tea that will assist with kicking cramp's ass! There is even an option to add a Delta-8 shot that will leave you feeling relaxed and discharged from any worries. Again, I recommend you proceed with caution and educate yourself thoroughly if you choose to use this form of herb for aesculapian purposes.

Chapter 7

We Are Made from Spice and Everything Nice

"Regarding the significant effect of cinnamon on reduction of pain, menstrual bleeding, nausea and vomiting with primary dysmenorrhea without side effects, it can be regarded as a safe and effective treatment for dysmenorrhea in young women." Jaafarpour, Hatefi, Najafi, Khajavikhan, & Khani. (2015)[7]

Are little girls really made from sugar, spice and everything nice?! Spices are vital not only in womb rejuvenation but overall health as they are imperative healing agents. Black Pepper has an active ingredient called piperine that increases the absorption of curcumin (active ingredient in *Turmeric* mentioned earlier) by 2000%. This spice also has anti-inflammatory properties, and antioxidants that offer pain relief and boosts absorption of nutrients.

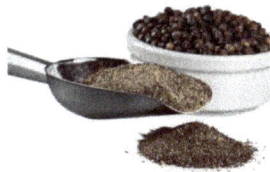

[7] Jaafarpour, M., Hatefi, M., Najafi, F., Khajavikhan, J., & Khani, A. (2015). The effect of cinnamon on menstrual bleeding and systemic symptoms with primary dysmenorrhea. Iranian Red Crescent medical journal, 17(4), e27032. https://doi.org/10.5812/ircmj.17(4)2015.27032

☀ **NNG recommends consuming spices daily to activate the healing agents. Incorporating black pepper combined with turmeric in your daily diet reduces inflammation and pain in the body.**

Another spice that we recommend for daily consumption is cinnamon. From historical records unearthed as early as Ancient Egypt, this spice diminishes pain, regulates menstrual bleeding and reduces nausea. Cinnamon is essential for reducing discomfort in the body and boosting prevention measures from other uterine ailments such as PCOS (Polycystic Ovarian Syndrome), infertility, and fibroids. Whether in food or in a beverage, cinnamon is packed with healing abilities, such as:

- ⊙ Anti-inflammatory

- ⊙ Reduces PMS symptoms

- ⊙ Decreases menstrual bleeding

- ⊙ Eliminates nausea/vomiting

- ⊙ Anti-fungal

- ⊙ Antimicrobial

- ⊙ Packed with antioxidants

> "Caring for myself is not self-indulgence. It is self -preservation, and that is an act of political warfare."
> — Audre Lorde

Cinnamon has so many essential benefits for the body overall but it's extremely useful when tackling cramps on a monthly basis. Sprinkling some in your tea, smoothie or dish of your choice, it is easy to merge with your regimen. You will notice how radiant your skin will glow after incorporating cinnamon into your daily diet. Nutmeg is another spice that seems to be used more in baked treats and beverages during the U.S. holiday season versus on a frequent basis. This spice relieves stress, decreases pain, and regulates hormones; so, sprinkling some into your tea or food will be an added benefit for your body.

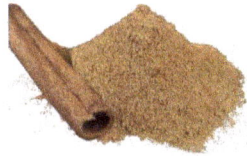

Chapter 8

Womb Revitalization

"Mugwort (Artemisia douglasiana) was, and still is, used to treat premenstrual syndrome and dysmenorrhea." (Adams & Garcia, 2006)[8]

I was introduced to the idea of yoni steams in 2018. This practice was new knowledge and I was enticed to learn more. Once I researched the healing powers that originated centuries ago, I was intrigued to see how it would work with my body. At first, I would only get steams annually, which changed to bi-annually. At one point, I was going every few months when I was located near a desired yoni spa. Talk about total womb revitalization! I am back to indulging annually, and I actually enjoy releasing these toxins and feeling sultry from the calefaction.

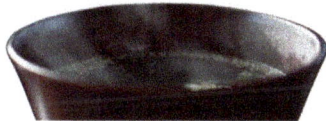

> ☀ **NNG recommends getting a yoni steam at least once a year.**

[8] Adams, J. D., Jr, & Garcia, C. (2006). Women's health among the Chumash. Evidence-based complementary and alternative medicine: eCAM, 3(1), 125–131. https://doi.org/10.1093/ecam/nek021

There are individuals who participate in monthly and even weekly steams. The herbs used in traditional steams were all mentioned in the ***Herbs*** section earlier. Many women are reluctant to sit over a hot pot of steaming herbs however, the benefits, and outcomes are vital for women's bodies. Below are the advantages of yoni steaming:

- ⊙ Tightens uterine walls
- ⊙ Reduces inflammation
- ⊙ Decreases pain
- ⊙ Cleanses access residue
- ⊙ Rejuvenates the womb
- ⊙ Regulates blood flow
- ⊙ Restores tissue walls
- ⊙ Boosts fertility
- ⊙ Repairs vaginal damage and tears
- ⊙ Prevents infections
- ⊙ Diminishes uterine health issues such as ovarian cysts, fibroids, PCOS or endometriosis

"The condition of women's wombs also directly reflects the condition of women's minds, spirits and actions. The womb is a storehouse of all of our emotions." — Queen Afua

There are many spas and wellness centers who now offer yoni steams; however, you can steam yourself at home as a DIY project! All you need is a wooden crate (with a hole in the top), a pot, herbs, and a blanket to cover up with. Buckets are easier to cut however be mindful of steaming plastic with not knowing where the material was generated or how many chemicals it may consume. Once you boil the herbs in a pot, you can set the pot in the bucket, place the top on then sit for 30 minutes with the bottom half of your body covered with the blanket. You can also get crafty with making a wooden box, cutting the applicable opening at the top to receive the steam and an entry to insert an electric pot, and a hole in order to plug it up. If you prefer to have back support then add a backrest, and even pad it if you want to get luxurious. Just be mindful if purchasing herbs or attending a spa, be sure that you research the reputability and the true knowledge the owner or specialist has on the yoni process. I highly encourage you to research yourself and follow your instinct on what works best for you. Mugwort, wormwood and calendula are my go-to main ingredients as a base for steaming. Mugwort tones and cleanses your vaginal walls by removing matter and energy. It also regulates and stimulates your hormones while protecting the womb from abnormalities. Wormwood provides anti-fungal and antibacterial healing components that rids yeast infections, Bacterial Vaginosis (BV), and undesirable discharge. Calendula drastically reduces inflammation and bloating while cleansing and soothing your womb from unwanted bacteria.

Chapter 9

Follow the Drip

In 40% of women, period pain is accompanied by premenstrual symptoms, such as bloating, tender breasts, swollen stomach, lack of concentration, mood swings, clumsiness and tiredness. (Women's Health Concern, 2022)[9]

Keeping track of your cycle is beneficial during your journey to kicking cramp's ass! Tracking the progression in your symptoms will allow you to forecast, and plan ahead, naturally. You may notice that your cycle may sync with the women you spend the most time with (best friend, mother, sister, coworker, etc.). Being a lesbian, it is common to sync with your partner; especially when you are on great terms. Who wants to deal with 2 raging, hormonal women grumbling about PMS symptoms at the same damn time?! Your menstrual cycle has 4 phases including menstruation, the follicular phase, ovulation and the luteal phase. Menstrual cramps and symptoms arise during the menstruation phase due to the previous cycle's eggs not being fertilized therefore, the uterus sheds its lining.

---

[9] Period pain. Women's Health Concern (2020, December 15). Retrieved February 22, 2022 from https://www.womens-health-concern.org/help-and-advice/factsheets/period-pain/

☀ **NNG recommends tracking all your uterine health outcomes as they arise.**

Factors that can be tracked includes menstrual cycles, symptoms, sexual activity, and even moods. There are many applications that you can download to track your period (some free and others offer subscriptions) such as:

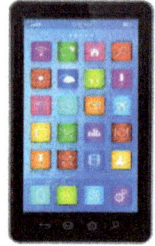

- ⊙ Period Tracker (what I have been using for years) - white background with pink flower as the logo
- ⊙ Flo
- ⊙ Clue
- ⊙ Glow
- ⊙ Period Tracker-Period Calendar (book w/ white flower as the logo)
- ⊙ My Calendar

In these trackers, you can maintain data on the items listed below plus more:

- ⊙ Start Date
- ⊙ End Date
- ⊙ Ovulation Day
- ⊙ Fertile Time Frame
- ⊙ When You Were Intimate
- ⊙ Nutrition
- ⊙ Medication
- ⊙ Water Consumption
- ⊙ Symptoms

- Moods
- Flow
- Notes
- Weight
- Conception Information
- Sleep
- Exercise

"I'm no longer accepting the things I cannot change. I'm changing the things I cannot accept."
— Angela Davis

Having a database where you can track what your body is craving, bloating, acne or tender breasts is essential. Monitoring your sexual activity is vital because if you have had unprotected sex, changed partners, or increase/decrease your activity, this can contribute to your menstrual cycle and cramp pain. Also, if you are sick or emotionally drained, you can notice an influx in your cramps therefore, having a tracker is extremely beneficial with kicking cramp's ass. Take time to follow the drip.

Chapter 10

Burrr - It's Cold in Here/It's Hot as Hell!

"This systematic review, which included six studies, found that heat therapy appears to decrease menstrual pain in women with primary dysmenorrhea." (Jo & Lee, 2018)[10]

Temperature control is most crucial during the first 2-3 days of menstruation. The body's climate tends to fluctuate while on your cycle due to the loss of blood. This correlates with iron anemia, as mentioned earlier in chapter 1. Now that you have established which tracking app you will be using, you can better monitor when your cycle will be starting. This will let you know how warmly, or hot flash-friendly, you should dress. The season and your location also play a role in determining how to best govern your body's temperature. "I said burr, it's cold in here!" So how are we going to kick cramp's ass with this method?!

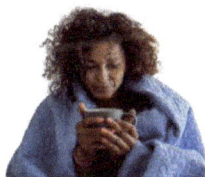

[10] Jo, J., & Lee, S. H. (2018). Heat therapy for primary dysmenorrhea: A systematic review and meta-analysis of its effects on pain relief and quality of life. Scientific reports, 8(1), 16252. https://doi.org/10.1038/s41598-018-34303-z

☀ **NNG recommends managing your temperature 2 days before the start of your cycle.**

If you have the tendency to cramp when you are cold, increase your body temperature by wearing long-sleeved clothing, pants/tights, socks, a hoodie or even wrapping yourself in an extra blanket. You better believe that I have my favorite cover to wrap up in (a plaid black, white and gray), socks (military combat footgear), hoodie (ranging from thick to thin based on the weather), and nightwear (long-sleeved vintage Victoria Secrets gown) that makes my cycle each month a breeze. Heat is a natural remedy for inflammation; so remaining warm during the menstruation process is essential. As mentioned in chapter 1, using a heating pad is the quickest way to warm yourself up. You have the luxury to place the heating pad in the area that is directly under distress. Another option for an at-home heating device is to make a rice sock. You heard that right! Throw some rice in a sock and place it in the oven for 1 minute. This does wonders; however, it will cool much quicker than anticipated. If you have the leisure of having seat warmers in your car, this makes your winters gratifying. Just be mindful that if you feel inflammation surfacing then implement a plan of action to regulate your temperature levels. Just do not overheat yourself then begin fanning and stating that, "It's hot as hell!"

"No! Of course, cramps don't hurt! It's just my body laying a freaking egg and if it doesn't get used, my body will just RIP down the wall inside me. No big deal." — Unknown

Chapter 11

Goddess Soak

"In an epidemiologic study of an adolescent population (age range, 12-17 years), Klein and Litt reported that dysmenorrhea had a prevalence of 59.7%. Of patients reporting pain, 12% described it as severe, 37% as moderate, and 49% as mild. Dysmenorrhea caused 14% of patients to miss school frequently." (Dong & Saski, 2021)[11]

Your cramping body + hot bath water = soothing sensations!

Taking a hot bath leading up to and during your cycle will not only rejuvenate your body but also suppress inflammation. Submerging your body in the water will regulate your body temperature; including Epsom salt or herbs can alleviate cramps due to their special healing powers, and better your overall mood. You can use the herbs stated in *Chapter 4: "Alchemy at its Finest" or* look into a special yoni blend. I actually like to use Beautiful Weirdos' *Mani Mix* which can be used in multiple cleansing techniques (more information in *Chapter 14: My Faves*). Hot baths also aid in reducing stress which is imperative in regulating menstrual

[11] Dong, A., & Sasaki, K. (2021). Dysmenorrhea. *Medscape*. Retrieved February 22, 2022 from https://emedicine.medscape.com/article/253812-overview

cramps. The less stress you endure, the more manageable your cycle will be.

I line the tub with my favorite crystals (Super Seven, 1 crystal for each chakra, plus some others!), chakra candles and will nourish myself with music, reading, writing or audio recording. Another frequent tendency is to rub on my waistbeads while basking in the restorative waters. If you are not aware, waistbeads enhances your femininity, spirituality, sensuality and fertility. Take a look at ancient African history; in the hieroglyphics, Goddesses wear waistbeads. It's embedded in our history, so why not participate in what has worked for centuries?! *eXccentricS* is who blesses my divinity with a plethora of waistbeads to choose from and educational material including what healing agents each color bead provides (you will discover more about these items also in *Chapter 14: My Faves*).

During the Goddess Soak, I tend to feel the most rejuvenated when I have completed my *Divine Rising Regimen*, which includes showing gratitude to the *Most High*, Universe and Ancestors, affirmations and manifestations through my vision board, meditate, reading at least 10 pages of the book of my choice (alternates between professional and pleasure reads), workout (toning the triple A's [Arms, Abs and Ass] or yoga), goal review, and calendar check. After getting in my Goddess zone, I can truly relax and exude the positive, productive and peaceful energy that was manifested. There's nothing like some self-love and care that we rightfully deserve; especially after putting up with the bullshit that menstruation can put us through every month. Channeling the beautiful African Goddess, *Oshún* takes me to an even higher frequency; as she has stopped a group of raging, menstruating women from taking over the world. With her power through water, it gives each of us rising Goddesses the opportunity to truly tap into our purity and how to love ourselves.

"A Nation can rise no higher than its Woman." — The Honorable Elijah Muhammad

☀ **NNG recommends soaking in the bathtub at least twice weekly for at least 30 minutes.**

Now this does not mean you cannot take baths daily because you are more than welcome to proceed with this method. With the busyness of our lives, we must relax to embark life back into our wombs. I typically like to take a bath the day before, day of, and second day of my cycle; it does wonders for my womb. The bath also provides the convenience to incorporate other self-care techniques such as exfoliating, milk bath bombs or another form of detoxing; especially if drinking freshly squeezed juice or tea. Either way, we are kicking ass arounds these kingdoms, dynasties or empires! Dancing a bit serenading myself as the water is filling the tub has become a component of this ritual maneuvering from African Goddess ritual dancing, Texas and Louisiana twerking or simply grooving to the beats that moves this physique. Remember you are beautiful and loved. It is important to remind yourself daily of the love you rightfully deserve; if you do not love yourself FIRST then it will be difficult to love anyone else, move on from past traumas or eliminate negative traits that hinder your transcendence. Accepting your worthiness and how you were made is applicable to your growth. You are everything and more, Goddess!

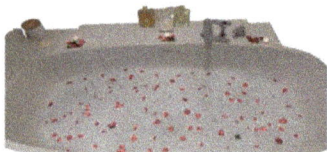

Chapter 12

I Keep HER Tight and Right!

"Some risk factors associated with primary menstrual pain are menarche at an early age, family history with menstrual pain, abnormal body mass index, the habit of eating fast food, menstruation duration, cigarette, coffee consumption, and psychological symptoms such as depression and anxiety." (Rahman, Hardi, Maras, & Riva, 2020).[12]

One of the most life changing moments I have had, is when I instantly saw results after changing the feminine hygiene products that I had been using my entire life. I think I was more baffled than anything to know that women around me including myself had been ignorant to the items that we were referred to for decades. Chemicals are the common denominator in all diagnoses! Be mindful whatever enters your vaginal hole goes directly into your bloodstream within a matter of minutes. Whether it is a childbirth defect, nutrient deficiency, mental health imbalance or simply an illness, it comes down to the amount of chemicals in

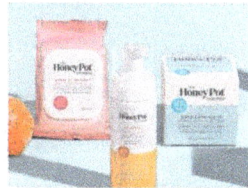

---

[12] Rahman, S. F., Hardi, G. W., Maras, M. A. J., and Riva, Y. R. (2020). Influence of Curcumin, and Ginger in Primary Dysmenorrhea: A Review. International Journal of Applied Engineering Research, 15(7), 634–638. Retrieved from www.ripublication.com.

your body, and the overuse, or lack of nutrients. So why eat foods made from chemicals, drink beverages full of toxins or wear feminine hygiene products that were made with these ingredients?! This aids in being odorless, preventing unnecessary discharge and regulating your menstrual blood color.

    ☀   **NNG recommends using and wearing all-natural and organic feminine hygiene products.**

I am a fan of trying different types of products as long as it contributes to positive health outcomes. I was never taught to not use bar soap on my vagina. WAIT A MINUTE! So, the times I went to the OB/GYN did she not plug me with the correct resources?! I used my very first yoni wash in 2018 from The Fem Expert (known as The Detox Girl, Lexi). It was like music to my vagina's ears! It not only drastically decreased my cramps, but also improved my overall vagina health. There's nothing like a fresh, plant-based vagina – the smell is impeccable! Lexi took a small hiatus which led me to other brands, *Garner's Garden*, *Goddess Body*, and *Femmagic*. I used the vagelixir from *Femmagic* one time and it truly deep cleaned the walls of my vagina; leaving a divine smell. Then I was introduced to *The HoneyPot Co* by Bea Dixon. First, let me say that I absolutely LOVE this woman's energy! In 2020, I had the opportunity to sit on a panel with her. She is always unapologetically herself and it was an honor to be in the presence of this Goddess! I currently use the original feminine wash (have tried the normal, sensitive, and cucumber aloe vera, which is my fave!), feminine wipes, and panty spray (I use this during the summer as this is a great alternative for natural armpits), and used to wear the pads before discovering the menstrual disc. On the days when I am not using their feminine wash, I use just water to clean my vagina.

Since starting my cycle, I used pads (all types), tampons (all types), menstrual cups, and discs. Tampons were my go-to in high school due to being an athlete but stopped using them in my late 20's as I had been diagnosed with Menorrhagia and could not keep up with the heavy flow of blood. Although tampons are cleaner than pads, once they are full then your body naturally starts to cramp because of the compacted area the tampon is placed in. So, after switching back to pads in 2016, it was much more comfortable although non-organic at that time for my cycle however it was a bloody mess (literally and figuratively!) In 2020, I attempted to use a menstrual cup, but it did not agree with my vagina at all. Immediately, I started using *The HoneyPot Co*'s pads, which I loved the tingling sensation that your vagina gets from the healing agents once you first put them on.

Then later that summer, I was introduced to the *Flex* menstrual disc by a midwife who had not used them yet. As I stated earlier, I am always open to trying new, effective products that will better my health, so I immediately purchased a box and started using them that night. This innovation is friggin' AMAZING! When I realized the minor cramps that would fluctuate from time to time had dropped from a 3 to a 1, on a 10-point pain scale. Although I love *The HoneyPot Co*, I made the switch (only for the pads, but I still use every product I mentioned above regarding *The HoneyPot Co.*) and have not turned back. At our consulting agency, we were blessed with a client named, *Vagesty* who is a melanin-owned business by a Women's Health Nurse Practitioner. She offers both disposable and reusable discs, in addition to other all-natural and organic feminine hygiene products, including period panties, subscription boxes, and women's health courses. Although the disc can take time to get used to, I could not ask for an even better product to wear while on my cycle. As I mentioned before, I prefer not to wear underwear and can put a disc in and go 12 hours with constant moving without any leakage or messes. You can "dump" by contracting your vaginal muscles when using the restroom; if you are afraid the disc is full. With an increase in sexual arousal while menstruating, you

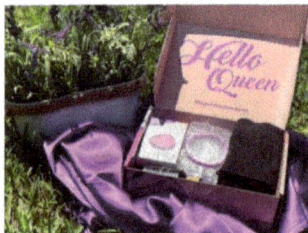

are also able to have sex with ease. You can discover more details during *Chapter 14: My Faves* on what we have used to keep HER tight and right during these case studies.

Other commons factors that contribute to keeping HER healthy are vaginal maintenance and sexual intercourse. Society has molded women to keep our genital areas free of hair and scold women who tend to live-out-loud naturally. Pubic hair helps defend your vagina from bacteria; its protective layer fights against vaginitis, urinary tract infections (UTIs) and yeast infections. The hair also safeguards the skin with moisture and reduces friction during sexual activities. Whether you shave, wax or sugar your vaginal hair, you must be aware of the chemicals in each product that are hazardous to women's health. Leftover residue can impact your pH balance resulting in unwanted odors, discharge or skin issues such as acne and ingrown hairs. Be intentional while caring for your vagina as we may groom to feel more sexually confident, however the ultimate goal is to avoid having cramps and negative health outcomes. If you are using products with perfume or scents that are chemical-based, it may take a toll on your health; just because it smells good does not mean it is the best option for your body. This also goes for regular perfume as well, Goddesses.

Some might say that sex is an extracurricular activity and fulfills your carnal desires (maybe it is just me!). Engaging in safe practices is **ALWAYS** recommended to avoid sexually transmitted diseases (STDs), women's health diagnoses, viruses or unplanned pregnancies. Once we, as women, allow an individual into our sacred space, we embody that energy and hygiene being projected from that individual. Having random sexual partners hinders your womb because it develops soul ties to frequencies that may keep your vibration low. If your body is purified and cleansed, in order to transcend to peaceful living, having sex with an impure, toxic person will contaminate your womb. No individual, sexual desire or temptation is worth the demise of your overall women's health! The yearn to be sexually pleased can be satisfied through a powerful manifestation masturbation where you are channeling your most divine self without the disturbance of negative energy seeking to leach from your transcendent being.

If after connecting with a new sex partner and if your cycle changes in any way, from the color, flow or symptoms, then this is the opportunity to review your menstrual tracking app and assess the changes accordingly. Protect HER at all costs and take accountability for what actions you take on this journey to optimal healing.

Unfortunately, there are many toilet paper brands that still add chemicals to their products. Why on earth would they need to add chemicals to an item that we have to use for multiple reasons whether we urinate, have a bowel movement or must wipe during our cycles?! Since we use toilet paper for everything, it would only make sense that over time those chemicals would obstruct the vagina and womb. After transitioning to a healthier lifestyle, bamboo toilet paper seemed to have the most sustainable and fresh approach to protecting HER.

In our *My Faves List* chapter, you can check out our recommended bamboo toilet paper option that has aided in kicking cramp's ass! This also goes for towels! Changing the towel you use on your vagina, body, and face are critical to keeping undesirable bacteria at bay. Your vagina cannot afford to absorb the germs from the remainder of your body. In the south, many of us were raised to use the same towel for some days before changing them. We (at least those around me) were not taught to have a separate vagina towel (only a full body and face). A wet towel that sits all day through various weather conditions accumulates so many germs and bacteria. You would be shocked if you examined a towel after the towel had set from 7:00am-7:00pm. And to think you saturate the towel in water, add more soap then place that bacteria back on to your vagina, body, and face. A quick fix to your pH balance and vaginal infections is to be deliberate with your vaginal maintenance. If you do not want to wash towels (yes, towels that are wet that have been sitting in the dirty clothes basket for weeks are crawling with bacteria every single second that passes by) daily then you can take it back to ancient history and wash yourself with your cleaned hands. Since towels aid in lathering of the soap, you may want to conduct this routine twice for a thorough restoration. As for your face, there are single-use towels available now; however, we keep a paper towel roll next to our face products so that we may pat dry the first round in our face regimen and throw the towel away immediately.

"When you replace "I" by "We," even illness becomes wellness."
— Malcolm X

Underwear, especially some nice lingerie is pleasant to have on deck. Victoria Secrets and I had a volatile relationship a decade or so ago because I kept a drawer full of sexy, intimate wear. G-strings, thongs, high waisted briefs, Brazilian cut panties - name them, I had them. Until I started this journey to defeat dysmenorrhea and cramps, I had not realized how much bacteria panties capture. If you have a fresh wax or shave, you want to avoid undergarments for chafing or developing hair bumps. While exercising, the panties are riding up your ass crack then possessing large amounts of sweat. You do not want a panty line so you wear a thong or G-string but may have discharge from the thin material cuffing your vulva leaving no circulation with the moisture that is growing. Too many back-to-back thong wearing leads to unwanted discharge. So why do we need underwear again? Perhaps to hold up your pad! Either way, if you choose to wear underclothing, change them frequently. After a long 8-hour workday (typically 11 hours if you include your to-from commute and lunch break), your vagina needs to breathe from being enclosed for almost half of the day. The buildup from sweat and other vaginal juices can lead to additional problems such as UTIs, yeast infections or unnecessary odors. Allow HER to breath after sex! Just how it is recommended to urinate after climaxing or having an orgasm, let that vagina exhale. Not buying new panties over time can leave unwanted bacteria festering if not washed immediately and with non-chemical laundry detergent. I particularly do not wear skivvies and have seen a tremendous change in my overall vaginal health since letting them go. I bet you are wondering what I do during my cycle. Those menstrual discs do wonders and leave me safe and confident with no leaking as I live out my active life! As we continue to eliminate the harmful factors that are hindering HER, we are closer to kicking cramp's ass and living a peaceful life with positive women's health outcomes.

Any product that you use, whether it is your toiletries or household products has an influence on your body. It is crucial that you use all-natural and all-organic products free from chemicals and toxins that overtime transition to various illnesses. Most people refrain from purchasing these products because they are expensive. With a growing environmental awareness industry, there are multiple items that are extremely affordable if you prioritize and budget accordingly. If you are a business owner or have a home office, purchase these items with OPM (other people's money) via business credit and it's a win/win. You not only enhance your health but also build business credit along the way while supporting eco-friendly organizations. If the business does not offer business credit directly, purchase these items from vendors (Amazon, Quill, etc.) who offer invoicing (NET-30, 60 or 90) or use a business retail card (Sam's Club, Walmart, Target, etc.) to make the purchase. With your toiletries, reconsider the toothpaste, mouthwash, bath soap, shampoo, conditioner, moisturizers or face products. Have you ever taken time to thoroughly read the ingredients in each product? If not, I challenge you to do so. For the ingredients that are foreign to you, research (use our handy dandy bestie, Google) what that item is and what harm it can do to the body. Educate yourself! Once you are more cognizant of what you are putting into your temple, you can make the best choices to avoid a health disturbance. The same goes for household products such as hand washing soap, laundry detergent or cleaning products as you should analyze what you are using. We as a society are so prone to do what the media, our families, and peers tell us to versus taking time to discover pertinent information for ourselves that will advance our welfare. Who cares if your Momo (aka grandmother) used a stellar house cleaning product! It does not matter if you have used the same soap on your face, body and vaginal area your entire life. Well, your T-Lady may have used those same pads because her mother and grandmother did, however that does not mean that those contents are best for you. Switch up your regimen and allow a few months to see realistic results on your overall health. Deodorant is a major debate with going natural! As a child, I did not comprehend the purpose of not wearing deodorant therefore was ignorant when it came to those who partook in this practice. I detoxed (did not wear any deodorant) for 1.5 years ridding myself of the *Secret* brand that has slid up and down my armpits for more than 2 decades. Was this a journey or what?! I now use the natural charcoal deodorant from *Garner's Garden* (I also used their tooth powder and mouthwash that turned my gums from extremely dark to a pure pink along with a plethora of other items outlined in chapter 16: *My Faves List)* however cleansing the body first was significant for removal of toxins. Why remove these chemicals? Because they are proven case studies that showcase the ingredients in certain deodorants are linked to cancer, Alzheimer's, dementia and kidney disease. Even swallowing tiny traces of toothpaste overtime may contribute to gastrointestinal disorders, nausea, weight gain, muscle spasms, and depression. Just because an item is approved by the FDA (Food and Drug Administration) does NOT mean it will protect you from the chemicals that we have our own eyes to read on every label. All that we ask is to be more conscious of the products that you apply now that you have been informed. Research the ramifications of these beauty techniques and products before diving in the deep end of a pool that may be hard to jump back out of after many years of damage to yourself. Fuck the peer pressure that society puts on us as women to showcase "what real beauty looks like!" One of my favorite moments of the day is expressing gratitude for the strength, courage, and wisdom to advocate for my health but also for the fine piece of specimen that Willie and Cal constructed! To have been such a superficial and vain individual in my teenage and second decade years, I wholeheartedly LOVE my natural beauty from the kink that flourishes from my crown's follicles to the melanin that is the impeccable shades of various earth tones (hints of golds, browns, reds, and oranges) to the body that I once was ashamed of and seriously hated to the diddy bop that these long legs migrate with. I accept every part of me and that's when you are at an optimal place of love and peace that you are ready to exude the same in healthy platonic and romantic relationships. I manifest that if you have not reached this level of frequency yet that it is in your near future!

Chapter 13

What You Put In and/or On Your Body Determines the REAL Fountain of Youth

"Age, family history, body mass index, socioeconomic status, education, smoking, and alcohol use can influence the severity of primary dysmenorrhea." (Bajalan, Alimoradi, Moafi, 2019)[13]

I cannot stress enough how important it is to be mindful of what you put in and/or on your body. During your cycle, you experience a loss of nutrients from your blood and need to replenish with the most nutritious forms of food. When I first became a chef, it was because I love to cater to others and see the look on their faces while they devour my delectable pieces of art. I put butter and heavy cream in damn near everything! It never occurred to me to cook to live versus cook to have the couch potatoes salivating at the television screen at one of my creations. Even when I was diagnosed with Diabetes, I did not resonate with the severity of my diagnosis because I was actively working out at that time, standing slightly under 5'8 and

---

[13] Bajalan Z, Alimoradi Z, Moafi F. (2019): Nutrition as a Potential Factor of Primary Dysmenorrhea: A Systematic Review of Observational Studies. Gynecol Obstet Invest 2019;84:209-224. doi: 10.1159/000495408

153 lbs. The diagnosis derived from the amount of sugar that I was putting in my body from the fruit juices made from concentrate, adding extra sugar to fruit drinks, excessive alcohol drinking and eating foods filled with sugar.

My lineage is from Texas, Louisiana, and Mississippi so adding "sugar water" to our watermelon to make it sweeter or 2-3lbs of sugar in our *Kool-Aid or Flavor Aid* was the norm. We always added extra sugar in our lemonade and Kool Cups (frozen Kool-Aid in a styrofoam cup which I was always a fruit punch, lemonade and raspberry Flavor-Aid-mix type of chic) because it tasted better. In blazing hot Texas or Louisiana summers, sucking on these bad boys, or the Bugs Bunny treat from the ice cream man, I did not realize how much poison I was ingesting as a child. All this sugar consumption accumulated overtime into a chronic illness that led to the death of my favorite grandfather. I would watch him hide desserts and treats in his office not realizing the cruelty he was inflicting on his body. The day after my 15th birthday, he passed away from kidney failure from his ongoing Diabetes. That day changed my life forever as I lost my hero. In 2014, the denial had reared its ugly little head and I would not be faced with how Diabetes started affecting me until I went from a size 6 to a 16W in less than 2 years after my diagnosis. *Disclaimer: I am not saying there is anything wrong with a size 16 but for ME personally, it made me uncomfortable, with weak knees, a* *double chin, development of dark spots in unwanted areas and nobody told me about the thigh acne!** My right eye became blurred therefore I had to begin wearing glasses, my left arm constantly tingled and I would lose feeling in my left hand, arm, leg, and foot frequently.

Throughout my life up until this point, which is now 2017, I had been diagnosed with so many other illnesses including Bipolar II Disorder, Irritable Bowel Syndrome (IBS), Viral Meningitis, Ovarian Cystitis, Acute Bronchitis, Menorrhagia, Dysmenorrhea, Allergic Rhinitis plus common colds, flus, stomach viruses, etc. Even as time went on, it still had not registered that diseases could be coming from the food or drinks that I consume let alone any of the products that I use on my body on a daily basis. As mentioned in the introduction of this book, I transitioned to a Vegan lifestyle on August 13, 2017, in an effort to lose weight for an upcoming life event. I did not realize how my life changed forever that day and each passing day that I am blessed to reign in this lifetime. Within a 3-month period, I lost 33lbs and started seeing a significant change. Then by the 8-month mark, I had stopped taking medication and had transitioned ALL of my toiletries (was already using natural hair products but started using all-natural and organic toothpaste, mouth wash, body shop, body moisturizer and deodorant). By the 1.5-year mark, I had changed my make-up, toilet paper, paper towels, hand soap, dishwashing soap, laundry detergent, fabric softener and household cleaning products. Then only used glass or bamboo options for cooking, eating, etc.

The moral to this story is to get rid of anything that has chemicals, toxins or genetically modified objects (GMOs). This includes eliminating processed foods such as fast food and canned goods. Majority of the foods that are white are highly processed and have been stripped of their real nutrients. These foods include white rice, white flour, granulated or powdered sugar. Added sugars (meaning not naturally from a fruit) or items made from high corn fructose syrup or concentrate are to be avoided as well. These items overtime will begin to develop into disease, accumulated mucus, unwanted chemical reactions, visceral fat (stubborn belly fat) and you guessed it, horrible menstrual cycles. Have you ever wondered why multiple people in your family gets the hereditary Cancer? Or why the women have horrible menstruation, yet they all know how to make the best oxtails, macaroni & cheese, and banana pudding? It is because we are repeating the same habits that lead to negative health outcomes. Even if you are in denial and do not want to believe the food and products that we are utilizing are slowly aiding in the demise of our health, you must take a step back and do your research. Have a conservation with the elders on some of the techniques that have been mentioned throughout this literature. If she has not participated in any of the methods, then why not try it for yourself to see what progress you can potentially make?

Eliminating unnecessary mucus from the body will slowly start to decrease the buildup of disease, onsetting viruses and other issues that will begin to impede the body. You can tell when hindering mucus has completely left the body because you will not experience sickness as frequently (not even common colds unless you come into contact with an individual with a weakened immune system), body odors will not be as strong, lose weight in areas that are difficult to shed, clear skin, and improve brain function due to the equilibrium in chemicals reactions. Also eating all the food groups daily (plant protein, complex carbohydrates, healthy fats, a variety of colorful vegetables, a variety of colorful seeded fruits, whole grains, herbs, nuts, and seeds) along with drinking plenty of water will provide your body with the applicable nutrients needed to sustain and add life longevity to your timeline. Incorporating probiotic foods, such as pickled vegetables or miso, will fight against inflammation and maintain a healthy pH balance. Items like red meat, caffeine-based, and alcohol have high amounts of carcinogens, toxins, and other chemicals that aids in inflammation and the onset of chronic illness such as heart disease and cancer. I

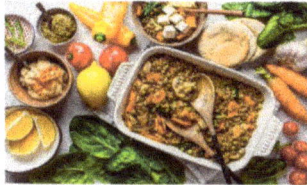

often get questioned on why not consume fish or seafood. Real simple - I am not trying to eat anything out of the ocean, especially in the Gulf of Mexico where there has been an abundance of spilled oil, waste, animal feces, plastic, and other toxins, that fish and sea creatures ingest then we eat them. Before transitioning to plant-based living, I was a huge fan of eating crawfish. How can I have both Creole and Cajun traits yet not want to devour some crawdaddies or grilled red snapper?! But after you sit and research the evolution and current environmental states, why would I subject my Goddess body to eating these tainted items?! Overtime, do you not think the crud from the ocean will not accrue into something that has been lingering and festering in your body for years? And do not get me started with how meat manufacturers cut the cancer off beef, pork and chicken then still turn around and sell it to the masses. Many of these poor cows have machines connected to their breasts controlling their pumping so the overworking of their nipples causes blood and puss to enter milk products in which the world is steadily consuming. Eating foods from reputable resources free of chemicals and toxins is the way in! I am walking around free of disease, and it feels great! Coming from the sickly child that stayed in the hospital or doctor's offices off and on for over a decade then grew into an adult that has developed even more diseases all because my body was beginning to reject the damage that I kept inflicting on her.

"I think the lack of critical engagement with the food that we eat demonstrates the extent to which the commodity form has become the primary way in which we perceive the world."
— Angela Davis

My recommendation is to take all your favorite food dishes and eat those in a plant-based form. This will make the transition much smoother and allows you to better acclimate to holistic living. It was a total culture shock when I went plant-based because it was an impulsive move. Cold turkey and never looked back. I literally ate French fries and salad (which I am not the biggest salad eater as my body metabolizes it fast leaving me hungry soon after eating it) for a little over a week not realizing how much I really had given up eating. "*What the Health*" definitely put into perspective what I had been doing to my body yet the idea of my illnesses reversing was still a figment of my imagination until a few months later when the case studies began. A trip to New Orleans was scheduled for 12 days later and the feeling of disbelief set in as I realized this meant no more red beans and rice (my favorite dish FYI!), no more *Mother's*, no more *Cafe du Monde*, no pecan pralines, no gumbo how I prefer, no crawfish with andouille sausage, potatoes and corn saturated in Cajun garlic butter, and no more of my favorite LGBT brunch spot, *The Country Club*. My heart sunk and I began to ponder how would I navigate as a vegan in NOLA.

"What am I going to eat?!"

"Can I survive in NOLA being Vegan?!

"What was I thinking to make this type of decision knowing I had this trip planned?!

As the fear and doubt began to roll in, it set in to look up Vegan options. At the time, I was residing in Katy, Texas, which is a suburb in northwest Houston, so if I wanted to eat the better Vegan options without having to cook, I would have to travel 45 minutes or so into the city. Since then (remember this was back in 2017), Katy has more options to choose from, however NOLA is much smaller than Houston so the options may not be more accessible is what I thought. Multiple options began to pop up and the place that captured my eye immediately was *Seed*. OH-MY-GOODNESS (In my Sheneneh Jenkins voice from *Martin*)! As soon as I saw their version of crab cakes, gumbo, and beignets, any fear and doubt, that attempted to knock me off my pedestal had dissipated. At the time, I was still drinking, so I engaged in my poison of choice, whisky. I must admit everything was extremely delectable! So damn good that it was made from a combination of Oshùn (African Goddess of the River of Beauty & Love) and Yemaya's (African Goddess of the Ocean of Motherly Love) tears! I was more than satisfied and it ignited a passion that I could take my culture's favorite dishes and veganize them. At least I would start doing that at my restaurant that I owned was the idea until Hurricane Harvey hit. This left me stranded in NOLA for longer than expected so I had the opportunity to explore pretty much every Vegan option they had available.

Nirvana was another favorite during this time, which I have always loved Indian food so bye Vindaloo, and hello Bhindi Masala (Punjabi style in a tomato sauce is BOMB.com) with Daal on the side. As time went on and I became more educated on vegan dishes, the transition to plant-based occurred steering away from overly processed vegan foods that can still lead to disease and focusing on the rawest form of a food item to gain the best nutrients. Curiosity from my maternal grandmother's chronic health diagnoses, my entire family's medical history, and the love I had for culinary led me to pursue a degree in Nutrition Education to determine how in the hell can I save my culture!

My entire career up until this point completely shifted and I now wanted to serve in a different form. I wanted to serve, heal, and educate the masses on how they too can start saving their lives. That is by being fulfilled in your optimal health. Optimal health for me includes your mental, emotional, spiritual, physical, and financial states. If you are consuming whole nutrients that aid in healing the body and maintaining positive chemical reactions in the brain, then this will assist multiple states. Your mental state is more manageable even if you must seek assistance from a therapist, counselor or life coach. If you are not adding any chemicals or toxins that can hinder your brain's function then your brain can remain at an equilibrium until it has a negative reaction, which can be handled through holistic tools and techniques from a reputable professional. Those same nutrients will assist with your emotional state with helping you to balance your mood and be accountable for your own actions, which you only control YOU in that very moment.

When your body is pure and cleansed, you become more in tune and connected with your highest spiritual form. No matter if you are spiritual or religious, both showcase detoxing, cleansing, fastening, and consuming clean foods will bring you closer to your highest frequency. We have briefly touched on physical activity and will talk a bit more about it soon. However, nutrient's main goals are to develop, preserve and restore all areas within the body. This includes supplying energy, the maintenance of the structure, and regulation of the chemical reactions in your body. Activating your neuromelanin ($C_{18}H_{10}N_2O_4$) with an ample amount of Vitamin D from the sun combined with legitimate nutrients (plant protein and water) will keep you powerful Goddess! And financially, that's where my entrepreneurial expertise comes in educating on building generational wealth.

The prior years of experience with nutrition education to my personal chef clientele and newly generated case studies were the foundation to what you have ingested from this book so far and what still is to come. As the diseases began to disappear, vision became corrected, weight fell off, mucus cleared out -

my brain unfolded how patience, discipline, knowledge, productivity, and consistency can truly save our lives. It will leave us peaceful. My purpose at that very moment was activated...

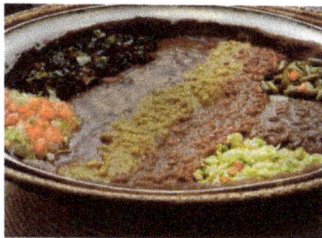

☀ **NNG recommends nourishing yourself by eating a plant-based diet daily.**

I would be fabricating if I say that I had not thought about meat ever again. Mainly crawfish, *WingStop* flat Cajun wings or my parents cooking me oxtails for my birthday, which haunted me the first couple of years around crawfish season or my birthday in October. But I love my body and my optimal health more! Food is truly medicine for the body. The feeling of not having to suffer year in and year out with the illnesses and medications I had to endure is exhilarating. Do you realize how much money you save being plant-based?! People will attempt to discourage you about how expensive it is because it can be if you are buying high market valued items. However, I can spend $45 for an entire week's worth of groceries and that's breakfast, lunch, dinner, snacks, and drinks. Then with the money I am saving on co-pays, deductibles from procedures, medications, and gas going to the doctor's office all the time does wonders for my pockets and wealth building. Going out to eat can get expensive but I was paying the same if not more when I would eat at a fine dining restaurant with a bottle of wine or 2 premium cocktails so what's all the fuss about?! I choose when to go out to eat and ensure that I am getting everything that I am craving if I am paying to be served. If I have not done so yet, I apologize to my body for not showering you with godly love but now that I am no longer ignorant to what I am exposing you to, I cherish and will treat you more exceptional than I have ever before. Your body is truly a temple and what you do to her now will determine what will happen in years to come. *"What you put in/or on your body will determine your path to the REAL Fountain of Youth!"* Now that we all know better, let's do better!

MICRONUTRIENTS - WHAT WE NEED IN SMALL DOSES

VITAMINS & MINERALS

There are various forms of vitamins and supplements that can ensure you are meeting the daily recommended value. Beware of the capsules as they are made from gelatin, animal fats and chemicals all associated with chronic illnesses. Beneficial supplements includes sea moss, spirulina, moringa and chlorella all provides reputable sources of vitamins and minerals. Consuming a wide variety of different colors of fruits and vegetables and tapping into each food group will aid in acquiring the micronutrients that the body needs.

Collards, mustards, kale, spinach, cabbage, bell pepper, okra, zucchini, asparagus, Brussel sprouts, broccoli, arugula, celery, cucumber, string beans, kiwi, apple, grape, lime, honeydew, pear

Squash, corn, potato, bell pepper, pineapple, mango, banana

Tomatoes, bell peppers, onions, potatoes, berries, apple, watermelon, cherries

Carrots, sweet potatoes, bell peppers, pumpkin, papaya, oranges, cantaloupe, peaches

Eggplant, cabbage, grapes, figs, currants, elderberry, plum, prunes

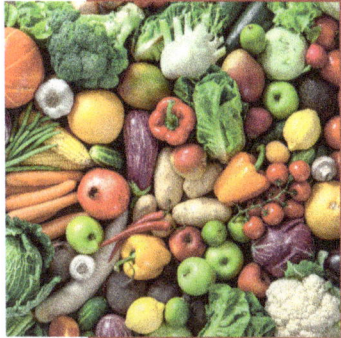

MACRONUTRIENTS -NUTRIENTS THAT WE NEED IN AN ABUNDANCE

PROTEINS

- Legumes (chickpeas, lentils, beans & peas)
- Leafy Greens (kale, collard greens)
- Mushrooms
- Quinoa, Wild Rice
- Seeds (hemp, pumpkin, flax, chia)
- Nuts (cashews, walnuts, pecans, hazel, macadamia)
- Tef, Splet
- Oatmeal
- Soy (tempeh, tofu, edamame)

CARBOHYDRATES

- Legumes (chickpeas, lentils, beans & peas)
- Potatoes (sweet, red)
- Whole Grains (quinoa, barley, oats, bread, cereal, pasta)
- Quinoa, Wild Rice
- Seeds (hemp, pumpkin, sesame)
- Squash (butternut, pumpkin)

FATS

- Avocado
- Tahini
- Seeds (hemp, pumpkin, sesame)
- Nuts (cashews, walnuts, pecans, hazel, macadamia)
- Cacao
- Oil (hempseed, grapeseed, coconut, olive, avocado, sesame)

SPICES: AVOID ADDED SODIUM, SEA OR HIMALAYAN IF YOU USE SALT, GINGER, TURMERIC, CINNAMON, CUMIN, CAYENNE, PAPRIKA, CHILI POWDER, CURRY, NUTMEG, HABANERO, SAFFRON, ROSEMARY, VANILLA

HERBS: THYME, BAY LEAVES, SAGE, BASIL, MINT, TARRAGON, OREGANO, DILL, CHIVES

TEA: BURDOCK, MOTHERWORT, NETTLES, RASPBERRY LEAF, HIBISCUS, GREEN, LEMON BALM, CHAMOMILE, GINGER, CALENDULA, ELDERBERRY

DRINK WATER DAILY (MINIMUM OF 8 CUPS PER DAY OR 4 (15.9 OZ) WATER BOTTLES)

OPTIMAL HEALTH TIPS

✓ Eliminate processed foods as it causes mucus build up in the body leading to disease, stubborn belly fat & obesity (anything white, bleached or with chemicals including fast food, canned goods, etc.)

✓ Avoid added sugar in food & beverages

✓ Drink **LOTS** of water & tea (decaffeinated)

✓ Indulge in fresh herbs through tea, food or steaming

✓ Exercise at least 5 days per week at a minimum of 30 minutes (even if it's only a 25-min yoga session including a 5-minute warm-up)

✓ Eliminate alcohol from the diet

✓ Incorporate ginger, turmeric and cinnamon into the daily diet

✓ Do **NOT** cook with oil. Cook with spring water **ONLY!**

✓ Avoid salt when possible and consume spices such as cumin, cayenne, paprika or curry

✓ Fresh squeeze juice **ONLY** (not from concentrate)

✓ Eat 3 times (breakfast, lunch & dinner) a day & 1 snack between 7:00am-7:00pm

✓ Sunbathing provides the best source of Vitamin D (and activates your melanin!)

✓ **ALWAYS** read the nutritional facts & ingredients on the back of food items

✓ Use all-natural and organic items including food, beverages, toiletries, household products, etc.

✓ Eliminate granulated sugar and use dates, raw sugar cane or organic raw agave instead

✓ Drink a minimum of 4 standard water bottles (15.9 oz) daily. 1 bottle per 3 meals & during 1 snack.

✓ Detox monthly (a minimum of 3 days). Consume raw foods **ONLY** for 2-4 weeks when completing a major detox in an effort to reverse chronic illnesses

✓ Indulge in positive mental health tools to avoid overeating or binge eating due to stress and anxiety

✓ Watch "What The Health?," "Seaspiracy," "Fork Over Knives," "Cowspiracy," & "Vegucated" to gain a better understanding of how food is handled in the United States & diseases that they cause

Chapter 14

Engaging in Some Extra Curricular Activity

"Severe pain sufficient to limit daily activities is considerably less common, affecting approximately 7%–15% of women, although a study of adolescents and young adults aged 26 years or less reported that 41% of the participants had limitations in their daily activities due to dysmenorrhea." (Hong Ju, Mark Jones, Gita Mishra, 2014).[14]

There is no quick and easy way around doing something that is worthwhile. With the pressure of society brainwashing us to believe that our bodies and appearance must be a specific way; we as women tend to get caught up in this superficial world. It took 4 years for me to transform to my desired muscle mass and health goals, and I strongly encourage you to put in the applicable work to get the results that you prefer. It takes patience, consistency and faith that you believe that you are capable of ANYTHING that you put your mind to. Nothing happens overnight and even if you use alternative options for losing weight, that will still not decrease your cramps or menstrual cycle symptoms if you are not proactively working out.

---

[14] Hong Ju, Mark Jones, Gita Mishra, The Prevalence and Risk Factors of Dysmenorrhea, *Epidemiologic Reviews*, Volume 36, Issue 1, 2014, Pages 104–113, https://doi.org/10.1093/epirev/mxt009

- ☀ **NNG recommends that you engage in physical activity at least 5 times per week at a minimum of 40 minutes daily.**

This may feel like it is a lot, but I am sure if you look at your "Screen Time" on your phone, it will show you are on social media longer than this time frame every day. You can even break the time into sections such as 5 minutes towards your warm-up, 15 minutes of anaerobic exercise (weightlifting, HIIT training, yoga, etc.), 15 minutes of aerobic exercise (running, brisk walking, cycling, etc.), and 5 minutes of cooling down. If you do not want to go to the gym or workout outside then there are plenty of apps on your phone, a plethora of videos on YouTube (I prefer Arianna Elizabeth with *Bright + Salted Yoga*, Juice & Toya with *One Body LA or Mrs. & Mrs. Muscle*) or programs through your cable, streaming or smart TV apps that will provide you with everything that you need to be consistent with your physical activity. These activities can be done as part of your "Start Your Day" regimen or in the evening before dinner. Feel free to increase your time and endurance overtime, and really watch your body heal and strengthen. I started working out every single day *Engaging in Some Extra Curricular Activity* with the following schedule:

- ⊙ Mondays, Wednesdays and Fridays: HIIT training, Body Sculpting Yoga and Walk/Run 2 miles (60-75 minute sessions)

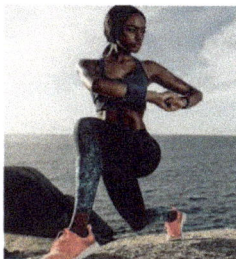

- ⊙ Tuesdays and Thursdays: Vizcaya Yoga, Ab workout and Walk/Run 2 miles (60-75 minute sessions)

- ⊙ Weekends: Restorative, and/or Deep Stretching Yoga, Ab workout and Walk/Run 2 miles (60-75 minute sessions)

  - None of the sessions include warm-up/cool down times
  - And ALWAYS completed after a session of showing gratitude to The Most High, Universe and Ancestors, meditation, and reviewing my vision board
  - You will only catch me running when I get to a beach so I can watch the sun rise and set while running along the perfect alignment (where Earth meets Water!) or in nature

"Be passionate and move forward with gusto every single hour of every single day until you reach your goal."
— Ava DuVernay

I often hear individuals say they cannot work out by themselves, or they need another individual motivating them to get the job done. In this world, you have full control of YOURSELF! Learning how to overcome obstacles by yourself not only makes you a stronger person but will allow you to no longer allow fear and doubt to interfere with your progress. What happens if that workout buddy cannot meet you today? Will you quit because s/he is not available, or will you push forward with your relevant goal?! Doing it all by yourself will empower you in ways that you never imagined so try it. Even when it gets hard, do NOT quit! Goddess, it WILL be worth it. Engaging in some extra curricular activity will not disappoint your body.

Chapter 15

Purified to the Fullest

"Results suggest that alcohol use premenstrually was related to the premenstrual symptom profiles whereas women whose alcohol use increased premenstrually had the highest premenstrual symptoms in areas of emotional well-being." (Carroll, Lustyk & Larimer, 2015).[15]

My name is Brittany, and I am an alcoholic...
I will never forget the day that I finally accepted this truth. It was February 2020, and my T-Lady stopped me in mid-conversation one afternoon and told me that I was an alcoholic. She mentioned that I talked about how many drinks that I had each day. In denial of course, I did not think that 3 extra strong whiskey sours or 3 glasses of pinot noir (really 7 cups because I would literally fill the 12oz red wine glass to the rim) every night was extreme. I mean, it was excessive to have these amounts after having dinner in a restaurant with 2 premium straight up and chilled Manhattans in my system. Or on the days I drove through the daiquiri shop during happy hour to get 3 extra shots for $1 in their largest size of their strongest drink. It is

---

[15] Carroll, H. A., Lustyk, M. K., & Larimer, M. E. (2015). The relationship between alcohol consumption and menstrual cycle: a review of the literature. Archives of women's mental health, 18(6), 773–781. https://doi.org/10.1007/s00737-015-0568-2

recommended that women only drink 1 cup of alcohol (2oz liquor with a mixer) or 1 glass of wine (5oz) daily. Leaving the conversation exasperated, I continued with my routine because I was not indulging in any illegal substances that led to rehab back in 2008 so what was the issue? Two months went by, and I endured so much stress from my full-time corporate job with major transitions (layoffs plus remote work training) due to the COVID-19 pandemic, my part-time position as a biology professor (also transitioned to 100% remote), a COO position of a non-profit catering to uterine health issues and battling many obstacles in my personal life. Overloaded was an understatement, yet I still managed to press forward and service all areas at 100% capacity leaving me to bask in my liquid pleasures every evening.

> "The eating of these chemicals [drugs, aspirin, depressants, amphetamines] indirectly causes robotized nutritional slavery (limits the range of thoughts and wellness)." - Dr. Llaila O. Afrika[16]

The case studies had proven that 90% of my cramps had disappeared. It was to the point that I could go several months without having a single cramp then out of nowhere, cramps would surface for only 1 month. I experienced this 3 times between the beginning of 2019 until the summer of 2020. On April 6, 2020, I went on an alcohol cleanse for 7 weeks. The goal was to go 60 days to break the habit of relying on

---

[16] Afrika, L. O. (2004). African Holistic Health. A & B Publishers Group.

alcohol to cope with what life was throwing my way. A mango margarita... that is what I drank that caused me to not meet my goals by 8 measly days. It was satisfying at the moment but the headache and nausea in the morning was out of this world. My body could never regurgitate however the nausea felt like a spiritual attack. Almost as if my soul was whimpering, "Why did you do this to us?!" After nourishing my body, the headache and abrogating feeling diminished. I went all week without a drink but decided the following weekend that I would indulge in a cup of wine. What do you know, I had another headache and the same gloomy feeling within my soul. Went another week without drinking then had a daiquiri the following weekend. Now this time, I did not have a headache, but the unfavorable sensation surfaced ten times! My body was literally so weak as if I contracted a virus. It had not resonated with what was really happening at this moment so of course, I continued about life. Went another week without alcohol then indulged in a rum punch from a restaurant that I frequently dined at. First thing in the morning, a mild headache and similar adverse reaction spiritually. The final week was near, and I took a trip to Austin for an event on June 27, 2020. Had a whiskey sour with *Maker's Mark*, however my body did not wait until the morning to quarrel but within 2 hours of consuming it, I was so ill that I could barely move. My head was spinning, and I kept feeling like I needed to heave but no food or liquid would eject. This would be the very last day that I take a sip of alcohol. My body kept talking but I was not listening. After having tequila, wine, rum, and whiskey over a span of a month and continued to get ill from each one. It was time for me to throw in the towel. I have always been surrounded by liquor whether it was a bar at my parent's house, a bar at my house after I moved out, at events because in our culture we love to eat and drink for any occasion. By the time that I was 22, I had a TABC, which allowed you to serve alcohol in Texas, so this tied in perfectly being a mixologist and a Chef. Alcohol is literally plastered everywhere in the media, restaurants and even tourist destinations. It saddens me when I hear individuals state they are bored so they will drink to fulfill their needs versus engaging in personal or professional development. I literally would steal liquor from my dad's bar in increments so I would not get caught and this was in middle school. After drinking consistently for 19 years, it felt good to say farewell to alcohol. At the end of the day, alcohol provides no nutritional value, is a chemical and toxin in addition adds sugar into the body. A quick way to get rid of that stubborn belly fat is to get rid of the booze. Or have you ever wondered how your mental health may continuously be impaired due to the amount of alcohol in your body? Just think about it, if you are mad and begin to drink, your emotions intensify. If you are sad and begin drinking, you may slip into a depression. When you add a chemical to an already imbalanced chemical state, this will only cause negative chemical reactions not providing any equilibrium to your brain functions. So again, what good is it that alcohol is really doing to the body?!

July 2020, no cramps. August 2020, no cramps. September 2020, no cramps. Here is where I experienced cramps every few months. October 2020, no cramps. November 2020, no cramps. December 2020, no cramps. Saying goodbye to alcohol finally provided that 10% that I was missing to kick cramp's ass for good. 2021 was my first complete full year of not having a single cramp. Even when inflammation was at a 2 on a scale of 1-10, either my body temperature was off, or I was overly stressed about a recent matter. Either way, it never resulted in cramps and was easy to get rid of by regulating my temperature and using positive mental health tools to eliminate unwanted anxiety and stress. For those of you who suffer from endometriosis, PCOS, infertility or other uterine health diagnoses, have you ever tried speaking to someone who holistically healed themselves from these illnesses? The first thing the Goddess will do is advise what she let go of in order to achieve victory over what has been troubling her womb. Unhealthy food choices, sugar, caffeine and alcohol is what I have heard consistently. As saturated as society portrays the importance of alcohol, it does not provide any

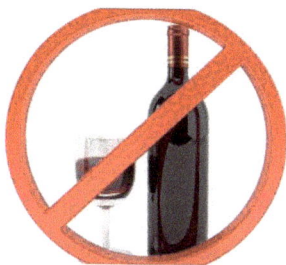

nutritional value and continues to burden our wombs. Yes, the contents make us feel good, aids in self-medicating and may give us liquid courage. However, those problems will still be there once you sober up. Once we no longer feel buzzed from the temporary although sometimes fun fix, do you have the ability to make yourself happy without a substance for assistance? Wouldn't you want to have the tenacity to always speak YOUR truth besides hiding behind a co-dependent factor? Even if you truly enjoy liquor and do not need it for any of the above-mentioned reasons, does it have more pros versus cons when evaluating the positive health advantages?! Another aha moment now that you know more about what could be possibly supplying your agony. What will your next move be?! *Purified to the Fullest* and it feels so good!

Chapter 16

My Faves List

"Some tampons are manufactured using harmful materials, including dioxin and pesticide residues. (Campaign for Safe Cosmetics, 2022)[17]

It would not be right if I did not let you in on which products I use to keep kicking cramp's ass! I mentioned most of these items or brands throughout the book. You will also see references and resources that will be beneficial as you are making the applicable changes to diminish your menstrual cramps. Be mindful that I am a firm believer of supporting the underrepresented so I will **ALWAYS** purchase from people of color **FIRST** in order to circulate melanin dollars. If what I need is not produced by a person of color, then I buy from a woman **SECOND**. Still searching for my desired product or service I then will purchase from a LGBT+ business. Being that I am all 3, it is always a pleasure to encounter individuals who meet 2 or 3 of the underrepresented categories.

---

[17] *Cumulative exposure and feminine care products.* Safe Cosmetics. (n.d.). Retrieved February 22, 2022, from https://www.safecosmetics.org/get-the-facts/healthandscience/cumulative-exposure-and-feminine-care-products/

Garner's Garden

- ⊙ All-Natural and Organic Toiletries
- ⊙ New Nation Goddess uses:
  - Shea Butter (Unscented and Lavender)
  - Natural Charcoal Deodorant
  - Mouthwash
  - Charcoal and Neem Tooth Powder
  - Aloe and Calendula Body Soap
  - Hand Moisturizer (Ginger)
  - Chapstick (Citrus)
  - Sanitizer
  - Body Oil (Citrus)

The HoneyPot Co.

- ⊙ All-Natural and Organic Feminine Hygiene Products
- ⊙ New Nation Goddess uses:
  - Feminine Wash (have used all but Cucumber Aloe [the original formula] is my favorite!)
  - Feminine Wipes (have used all but Cucumber Aloe [the original formula] is my favorite!)
  - Pantry Spray (original lavender formula - for armpits during the summer)
  - Panty Liners (if you happen to spot and do not want to use a menstrual disc)

Reel

- ⊙ All-Natural and Organic Bamboo Toilet Paper
- ⊙ New Nation Goddess uses:
  - Toilet Tissue

The True Products

- ⊙ All-Natural & Organic Laundry Products
- ⊙ New Nation Goddess uses:
  - Laundry Detergent (Sensitive Skin)
  - Fabric Softener (Sensitive Skin)

Naturaleza's Apothecary

- ⊙ All-Natural & Organic Face & Skin Care
- ⊙ New Nation Goddess uses:
  - *"Show Your Glow"* Collection
    - Cleanser
    - Toner
    - Serum
  - *"Fountain of Youth"* Serum
  - Quintessential Body Moisturizer

Vagesty

- ⊙ All-Natural & Organic Feminine Hygiene Products
- ⊙ New Nation Goddess uses:
  - Disposable Menstrual Discs
  - Feminine Wipes

Beautiful Weirdos

- ⊙ Metaphysical Treasures
- ⊙ New Nation Goddess uses:
  - Mani Mix (perfect for herbal baths or in candles for new moon/full moon rituals or even your daily affirmation/manifestation regimen)
  - Crystal Pendants
    - Carnelian (one of my faves which channels creativity)
    - Selenite (My FAVE! - represents big dick energy)
    - Lapis Lazuli (represents communication)
    - Amazonite (aids in maintaining optimal health)
    - Jasper Agate Arrowhead (represents tranquility, wholeness and offers protection)
    - Incense

Flex

- ⊙ All-Natural and Organic Feminine Hygiene Products
- ⊙ New Nation Goddess uses:
  - Disposable Menstrual Discs

eXccentricS

- ⊙ Metaphysical Store
- ⊙ New Nation Goddess uses:
  - Waistbeads
  - Bookmarks (customizable)
  - The Sage Vault (custom crystal carrier which houses ALL of my crystals including my favorite, a Super Seven! Mines is customized with my favorite colors and birth chart)

You can purchase from the resources listed and receive dollars or percentages off select items by scanning this code

Additional Resources

Books

- "Sacred Woman" by Queen Afua
- "Heal Thyself" by Queen Afua
- "African Holistic Health" by Dr. Llaila Afrika

Organizations

- Black Women's Health Imperative
- Afro Vegan Society
- Love Your Menses
- Endo Black
- National Black Doulas Association

Experts

- The Fem Health Expert Lexi, Wellness Coach
- Dr. Janelle Howell, Pelvic Physical Therapist
- Adrienne Brown, Sex Therapist
- Iesha Anderson, New Beginning Mind Spa and Therapy, Licensed Professional Counselor
- Arianna Elizabeth, Bright and Salted Yoga, Yoga Instructor
- Juice & Toya, One Body LA, Fitness Trainers
- Mr. & Mrs. Muscle, Fitness Trainers

Documentaries/Films

- What the Health?
- Seaspiracy
- They're Trying to Kill Us
- Forks Over Knives
- Vegucated

Chapter 17

Nutrition Consultation Information

New Nation Goddess, Inc. is here to serve you POSITIVE, PRODUCTIVE and PEACEFUL strategies! We offer nutrition consulting (and business if needed) services to individuals, assisting them to achieve optimal wellness. If you have any questions or concerns regarding any of the information located within this book, feel free to contact us so that we may better serve you. You can schedule a consultation by scanning this code:

FLOWCODE

PRIVACY.FLOWCODE.COM

Chapter 18

Menstrual Blood Chart

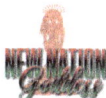

HEALTHY PERIOD

LIGHT BLEEDING
POTENTIALLY LOW ESTROGEN LEVELS NUTRIENT
DEFICIENCY
PERIOD BLOOD MIXED W/ VAGINAL FLUIDS

VAGINAL INFECTION
BLOOD MIXED WITH CERVICAL FLUID

HIGH ESTROGEN
VAGINAL INFECTION
BLOOD MIXED WITH CERVICAL FLUID
HEAVY BLEEDING
SYMPTOM OF OVARIAN CYSTS, PCOS OR
ENDOMETRIOSIS

BLOOD FROM PREVIOUS CYCLE
LOW PROGESTERONE

BACTERIA VAGINOSIS

Chapter 19

Womb Manifestations

"I AM" Statements = Inspiration, Affirmations and Manifestations

- ★ **I am a GODDESS!**
- ★ **I am PEACEFUL!**
- ★ **I am DIVINE!**
- ★ **I am WORTHY!**
- ★ **I am VALUABLE!**
- ★ **I am BEAUTIFUL!**
- ★ **I am FEMININE!**
- ★ **I am STRONG!**
- ★ **I am WEALTHY!**
- ★ **I am FOCUSED!**
- ★ **I am UNSTOPPABLE!**
- ★ **I am grateful for my body!**
- ★ **I am appreciative of another opportunity in life!**
- ★ **I am healing myself!**

★ I am achieving optimal health!

★ I am transcending to my highest frequency!

★ I am accepting the knowledge and gifts from the Most High, Universe and Ancestors!

★ I am obtaining knowledge to define my purpose!

★ I am revitalizing my womb!

★ I am setting applicable boundaries to protect myself!

★ I am eliminating stressful situations!

★ I am in love with myself & giving self-love on a frequent basis!